NAVIGATING THE USE OF MIFEPRISTONE

THE COMPREHENSIVE GUIDE ON THE APPLICATIONS AND SAFE ADMINISTRATION FOR EARLY PREGNANCY TERMINATION

TABLE OF CONTENTS

CHAPTER 1

INTRODUCTION TO MIFEPRISTONE

1.1 Overview of Early Pregnancy Termination

Early pregnancy termination, also known as abortion, is the process of ending a pregnancy during its initial stages, typically within the first trimester. This period, which lasts up to 12 weeks of gestation, is crucial for many women who, for various reasons, decide not to carry the pregnancy to term. The reasons for early pregnancy termination vary widely and can include personal, medical, social, or economic factors. Some women might face health risks if the pregnancy continues, while others might not be prepared for the responsibilities that come with raising a child.

Early pregnancy termination can be achieved through different methods, broadly categorized into surgical and medical options. Surgical methods, such as vacuum aspiration, involve physically removing the contents of the uterus. These procedures are typically performed in clinical settings by healthcare professionals. On the other hand, medical termination involves the use of pharmaceutical drugs to induce abortion. This method has become increasingly popular due to its non-invasive nature and the possibility of being administered in more private settings.

One of the most commonly used methods for early pregnancy termination is the administration of a combination of two medications: mifepristone and misoprostol. Mifepristone, also known as RU-486, plays a central role in this medical regimen, offering a safe and effective option for women seeking to end a pregnancy during the first trimester. Its development and use have revolutionized the approach to early pregnancy termination, making it more accessible and acceptable worldwide.

1.2 What is Mifepristone?

Mifepristone is a synthetic steroid that functions as an antiprogestogen, meaning it blocks the action of progesterone—a hormone essential for maintaining pregnancy. By binding to the progesterone receptors in the body, mifepristone effectively disrupts the hormonal support required for the continued growth of the embryo. This action makes the uterine lining inhospitable, leading to the detachment of the embryo and the cessation of pregnancy.

Typically, mifepristone is used in combination with another drug, misoprostol, which induces uterine contractions to expel the pregnancy tissue from the uterus. This combination is highly effective, with a success rate of over 95% when used within the first 10 weeks of pregnancy. The process generally begins with the administration of mifepristone, followed by misoprostol 24 to 48 hours later. The procedure is considered complete once the pregnancy tissue is expelled, which usually occurs within a few hours after taking misoprostol.

The use of mifepristone in medical abortion has several advantages. It is less invasive than surgical methods, can be administered in an outpatient setting, and allows women more control over the timing and privacy of the procedure. Additionally, mifepristone has a relatively low side effect profile, with the most common effects being cramping and bleeding, similar to those experienced during a miscarriage.

1.3 History and Development

The development of mifepristone is a significant milestone in the history of reproductive health. The drug was first synthesized in 1980 by French scientist Étienne-Émile Baulieu, working with the pharmaceutical company Roussel-Uclaf. Baulieu's research focused on the role of hormones in pregnancy, leading to the discovery of mifepristone as a compound that could effectively block progesterone, a hormone crucial for the maintenance of pregnancy.

Mifepristone, initially known as RU-486, quickly garnered attention due to its potential use as a safe and effective method for terminating early pregnancies. However, its development and approval were met with considerable controversy, especially in countries with strong anti-abortion movements. Despite this, France became the first country to approve mifepristone for medical abortion in 1988. The French government recognized its potential for improving women's health and stepped in to ensure its availability despite opposition.

The approval of mifepristone in other countries followed, albeit at a slower pace. The drug faced significant political and social challenges, particularly in the United States, where it was approved by the Food and Drug

Administration (FDA) only in 2000 after years of debate and rigorous testing. The delay was largely due to concerns about the ethical implications of its use, as well as pressure from various interest groups. However, once approved, mifepristone became a cornerstone of medical abortion in the United States and many other countries.

Since its introduction, mifepristone has been used by millions of women worldwide. It has significantly changed the landscape of abortion services by providing a safe, effective, and less invasive option for early pregnancy termination. Research and development around mifepristone continue, with ongoing studies exploring its potential uses in other medical conditions, such as treating certain types of cancer and Cushing's syndrome.

1.4 Importance and Relevance

Mifepristone's importance in reproductive healthcare cannot be overstated. It has revolutionized the approach to early pregnancy termination by offering a safe, effective, and accessible alternative to surgical abortion. The drug has empowered women by providing them with more choices in managing their reproductive health and has helped reduce the stigma associated with abortion by enabling it to be performed in a more private and less invasive manner.

The availability of mifepristone has also had significant public health implications. In areas where access to surgical abortion is limited, either due to legal restrictions, lack of healthcare infrastructure, or social stigma, mifepristone provides a crucial alternative. It has been particularly important in low- and middle-income countries, where access to safe abortion services is often restricted, and unsafe abortion practices are a leading cause of maternal mortality. By offering a safer option, mifepristone has the potential to reduce the incidence of complications and deaths associated with unsafe abortions.

In addition to its role in abortion, mifepristone's potential uses in other areas of medicine continue to be explored. For instance, it is being investigated for the treatment of conditions like endometriosis, fibroids, and certain types of breast cancer, all of which involve hormonal regulation. Its ability to block progesterone makes it a valuable tool in these areas of research, offering hope for new therapeutic options.

Mifepristone remains a focal point in the ongoing debate over reproductive rights. Its use and availability are often challenged by political, religious, and social groups opposed to abortion. Despite these challenges, the drug has remained an essential component of reproductive healthcare in many parts of the world, underscoring the need for continued advocacy to ensure that women have access to safe and effective options for managing their reproductive health.

CHAPTER 2

HOW MIFEPRISTONE WORKS

2.1 Mechanism of Action

Mifepristone, also known as RU-486, is a synthetic steroid with a unique mechanism of action that makes it an effective option for medical abortion, particularly during the early stages of pregnancy. The drug works primarily by blocking the effects of progesterone, a hormone crucial for maintaining pregnancy. Progesterone is essential for the preparation and maintenance of the endometrium (the lining of the uterus), which supports the early stages of embryo development. Without the stabilizing effects of progesterone, the uterine lining begins to break down, leading to the detachment of the embryo and the cessation of pregnancy.

Mifepristone is classified as an antiprogestogen because it binds to the progesterone receptors in the body without activating them. By occupying these receptors, mifepristone prevents progesterone from exerting its effects on the uterine lining. As a result, the endometrium becomes unsuitable for sustaining the pregnancy, leading to the separation of the gestational sac from the uterine wall.

In addition to its antiprogestogenic effects, mifepristone also has a secondary mechanism of action that contributes to its effectiveness in inducing abortion. The drug causes the cervix to soften and dilate, which facilitates the passage of pregnancy tissue from the uterus. This cervical ripening effect is particularly important when mifepristone is used in combination with a prostaglandin analog, such as misoprostol, which induces uterine contractions.

When mifepristone is administered, it sets off a chain of physiological events. Within hours of ingestion, the progesterone blockade begins to affect the uterine lining, leading to its degradation. The embryo, no longer supported by a viable endometrium, detaches and stops growing. Mifepristone also increases the sensitivity of the uterus to the effects of prostaglandins, enhancing the contractions induced by misoprostol. These contractions help to expel the pregnancy tissue from the uterus, completing the abortion process.

2.2 Effectiveness

Mifepristone, when used in combination with misoprostol, is highly effective in inducing abortion during the first trimester of pregnancy. The effectiveness of this combination is well-documented, with success rates exceeding 95% when used appropriately. Several factors contribute to the high effectiveness of mifepristone-misoprostol regimens, including the timing of administration, the dosage, and the adherence to the recommended protocol.

One of the key reasons for the high effectiveness of mifepristone is its ability to thoroughly disrupt the hormonal environment necessary for sustaining pregnancy. By blocking progesterone, mifepristone ensures that the uterine lining cannot support the growing embryo, making the abortion process highly reliable. The addition of misoprostol, a prostaglandin analog that induces uterine contractions, further enhances the effectiveness of the regimen by ensuring that the pregnancy tissue is expelled from the uterus.

The standard protocol for medical abortion involves the administration of 200 mg of mifepristone, followed by 800 micrograms of misoprostol 24 to 48 hours later. This regimen has been extensively studied and has been shown to be highly effective for pregnancies up to 10 weeks of gestation. The success rate decreases slightly with increasing gestational age, but even at 10 weeks, the combination remains effective in the vast majority of cases.

In cases where the initial regimen does not result in a complete abortion, additional doses of misoprostol may be administered to enhance uterine contractions and complete the process. In rare cases where the abortion is incomplete or unsuccessful, a surgical procedure, such as vacuum aspiration, may be required to remove any remaining pregnancy tissue.

The effectiveness of mifepristone-misoprostol regimens has been validated through numerous clinical trials and real-world studies. These studies consistently demonstrate that the combination is not only effective but also safe for the vast majority of women. The side effects associated with the regimen, such as cramping and bleeding, are generally well-tolerated and are similar to those experienced during a natural miscarriage.

2.3 Time Frame for Usage

The time frame for using mifepristone in combination with misoprostol is crucial for ensuring the effectiveness and safety of the medical abortion process. Mifepristone is most effective when used during the first 10 weeks of pregnancy, with its efficacy being highest in the earlier weeks of gestation. The timing of administration within this window is guided by several factors, including the gestational age of the pregnancy, the patient's health status, and the specific medical protocol being followed.

Mifepristone is approved for use up to 70 days (10 weeks) of gestation. The earlier in the pregnancy that the medication is used, the more effective it tends to be. Studies have shown that the combination of mifepristone and misoprostol is over 95% effective when used within the first 7 weeks of pregnancy. As the pregnancy progresses, the success rate remains high but begins to decline slightly, with the effectiveness still remaining above 90% up to 10 weeks.

The standard regimen involves taking 200 mg of mifepristone orally, followed by 800 micrograms of misoprostol, which can be administered buccally (in the cheek), sublingually (under the tongue), or vaginally. The misoprostol is typically taken 24 to 48 hours after the mifepristone, allowing time for the drug to exert its effects on the uterine lining and cervical tissue. This two-step process is designed to maximize the effectiveness of the medication while minimizing the risks associated with the abortion process.

Beyond 10 weeks of gestation, the effectiveness of mifepristone begins to decrease, and the risks associated with the procedure increase. For pregnancies beyond this point, other methods of abortion, such as surgical procedures, are generally recommended. However, in some cases, medical abortion with mifepristone and misoprostol may still be considered under the guidance of a healthcare provider, with adjusted dosages and close monitoring.

The timing of administration is also important in the context of the patient's health and access to medical care. For women who have access to healthcare facilities, the standard 24- to 48-hour interval between mifepristone and misoprostol is usually recommended. However, in cases where access to healthcare is limited, or where the patient prefers to complete the process more quickly, misoprostol may be administered as soon as 6 hours after mifepristone. This shorter interval has been shown to be effective, although it may be associated with a slightly higher risk of side effects.

It is important to note that while the majority of women experience a complete abortion within a few hours of taking misoprostol, the process can sometimes take longer. In some cases, it may take several days for all the pregnancy tissue to be expelled from the uterus. Patients are typically advised to have a follow-up appointment with their healthcare provider 7 to 14 days after taking the medication to confirm that the abortion is complete and to check for any complications.

CHAPTER 3

USAGE GUIDELINES

3.1 Indications for Use

Mifepristone is primarily indicated for the medical termination of intrauterine pregnancy, particularly in the early stages. The drug is approved for use up to 10 weeks of gestation (70 days from the first day of the last menstrual period). It is commonly used in combination with misoprostol, a prostaglandin analog that induces uterine contractions, to increase the effectiveness of the abortion process. This combination is highly effective for women who are seeking to terminate a pregnancy without undergoing surgical procedures.

Mifepristone is also indicated for certain medical conditions outside of pregnancy termination. For instance, it is used in the treatment of Cushing's syndrome, particularly in cases where the condition is caused by an excess of cortisol. The drug works by blocking cortisol receptors, thereby reducing the effects of excess cortisol on the body. Additionally, mifepristone is being studied for its potential in treating other conditions, such as uterine fibroids and endometriosis, although its primary indication remains pregnancy termination.

Patients who are eligible for mifepristone typically include those who have confirmed pregnancies within the first 10 weeks of gestation and who prefer a medical over a surgical abortion. It is particularly indicated for women who seek a non-invasive, private option for pregnancy termination. However, the drug is contraindicated in certain cases, such as in women with ectopic pregnancies (where the embryo implants outside the uterus), chronic adrenal failure, or those who are on long-term corticosteroid therapy. Additionally, mifepristone should not be used in women who have an intrauterine device (IUD) in place unless the device is removed prior to administration.

3.2 Dosage Instructions

The dosage of mifepristone for the medical termination of pregnancy is standardized to ensure its effectiveness and safety. The typical regimen involves a single oral dose of 200 mg of mifepristone, followed by 800 micrograms of misoprostol, which is taken 24 to 48 hours later. This regimen is designed to maximize the efficacy of the medication while minimizing the potential for adverse effects.

The 200 mg dose of mifepristone is administered as a single tablet, which is taken orally with water. This dosage is sufficient to block the progesterone receptors in the body, leading to the breakdown of the uterine lining and the detachment of the embryo. The misoprostol, which is taken after the mifepristone, can be administered in several ways: orally (buccally, where the tablet is placed between the gum and cheek), sublingually (under the tongue), or vaginally. The route of administration for misoprostol may vary depending on the healthcare provider's recommendation and the patient's preference.

In some cases, healthcare providers may adjust the dosage or timing based on individual patient needs, particularly if the patient is further along in the pregnancy or has certain medical conditions. However, the standard 200 mg dose of mifepristone followed by 800 micrograms of misoprostol remains the most commonly prescribed regimen for early pregnancy termination.

For the treatment of Cushing's syndrome, the dosage of mifepristone is different and is tailored to the patient's specific condition. The starting dose typically ranges from 300 mg to 1200 mg per day, depending on the severity of the condition and the patient's response to treatment. The dose may be adjusted over time based on clinical response and the presence of any side effects.

3.3 How to Take Mifepristone

Taking mifepristone as part of a medical abortion regimen involves following a carefully structured process to ensure the effectiveness and safety of the procedure. The process begins with the administration of mifepristone, which is typically done in a healthcare setting, although it may also be taken at home under the guidance of a healthcare provider.

To take mifepristone:

1. **Confirm the Pregnancy**: Before taking mifepristone, it is essential to confirm the pregnancy through a reliable test, such as an ultrasound. This ensures that the pregnancy is within the appropriate gestational age for medical abortion and that there are no contraindications, such as an ectopic pregnancy.

2. **Consult with a Healthcare Provider**: A healthcare provider will assess the patient's medical history, current health status, and the specific circumstances of the pregnancy. This consultation helps to ensure that mifepristone is the appropriate choice and that the patient understands the process, potential side effects, and what to expect.

3. **Take the Mifepristone**: The patient takes a single 200 mg tablet of mifepristone orally with water. This dose can be taken in the presence of a healthcare provider or at home, depending on the patient's situation and local medical guidelines.

4. **Wait for 24 to 48 Hours**: After taking mifepristone, the patient must wait 24 to 48 hours before taking the next medication, misoprostol. During this time, the mifepristone works to block progesterone, leading to the breakdown of the uterine lining.

5. **Take Misoprostol**: After the waiting period, the patient takes 800 micrograms of misoprostol. This medication can be taken in various ways, depending on the patient's preference and the guidance of the healthcare provider. Misoprostol induces uterine contractions, leading to the expulsion of the pregnancy tissue.

6. **Follow-Up Care**: It is important to have a follow-up appointment with a healthcare provider 7 to 14 days after taking mifepristone and misoprostol to ensure that the abortion is complete and that there are no complications. This follow-up may involve an ultrasound or a physical examination.

Taking mifepristone is generally straightforward, but patients should be aware of potential side effects, such as cramping, bleeding, nausea, and fatigue, which are similar to the symptoms of a miscarriage. In rare cases, more serious side effects, such as heavy bleeding or infection, may occur, and patients should seek medical attention if they experience severe symptoms.

3.4 What to Do If You Miss a Dose

In the context of medical abortion, missing a dose of mifepristone is unlikely, as the drug is typically administered as a single dose under medical supervision. However, if a patient does not take misoprostol within the recommended 24 to 48 hours after taking mifepristone, it is essential to understand the potential implications and take appropriate action.

If a patient misses the scheduled time to take misoprostol after mifepristone, the following steps should be taken:

1. **Take the Misoprostol as Soon as Possible**: If the 24 to 48-hour window has passed, the patient should take misoprostol as soon as possible. While the standard interval is recommended to optimize effectiveness, taking the misoprostol a bit later may still result in a successful abortion, although the success rate may be slightly reduced.

2. **Contact a Healthcare Provider**: It is important to contact a healthcare provider to inform them of the missed dose and seek guidance on the next steps. The provider may recommend taking the misoprostol later than initially planned or suggest an alternative approach depending on how much time has passed.

3. **Monitor for Symptoms**: After taking misoprostol, the patient should monitor for the expected symptoms of cramping and bleeding, which indicate that the abortion process is underway. If these symptoms do not occur or if they are unusually mild, the patient should contact their healthcare provider, as this may indicate an incomplete abortion.

4. **Follow Up**: Regardless of when the misoprostol is taken, a follow-up appointment with a healthcare

provider is essential to confirm that the abortion is complete and that there are no complications. This appointment typically occurs 7 to 14 days after taking the medications.

In rare cases where a significant amount of time has passed without taking misoprostol, the healthcare provider may recommend repeating the entire regimen or opting for a surgical abortion to ensure the pregnancy is terminated effectively.

For patients using mifepristone for non-abortion purposes, such as in the treatment of Cushing's syndrome, missing a dose may have different implications. In such cases, it is generally recommended to take the missed dose as soon as it is remembered, unless it is close to the time for the next dose. In such cases, the missed dose should be skipped to avoid doubling up on medication. However, patients should always follow the specific advice of their healthcare provider in such situations.

CHAPTER 4

SIDE EFFECTS AND SAFETY

4.1 Common Side Effects

Mifepristone, when used as part of a medical abortion regimen, is generally well-tolerated, but like all medications, it can cause side effects. The most common side effects are related to the intended effects of the drug on the body. These side effects are generally manageable and are similar to the symptoms experienced during a natural miscarriage. They include:

1. **Bleeding**: Vaginal bleeding is the most common side effect of mifepristone. It occurs as the pregnancy tissue is expelled from the uterus. The bleeding may start as light spotting but typically becomes heavier after taking the accompanying medication, misoprostol. The bleeding can last for several days or even weeks, similar to a heavy menstrual period. In most cases, the bleeding gradually tapers off as the uterus expels the pregnancy tissue.

2. **Cramping**: Uterine cramping is another common side effect, resulting from the contractions of the uterus as it

expels the pregnancy tissue. The severity of cramping varies from person to person, with some women experiencing mild discomfort and others experiencing more intense pain. Over-the-counter pain relievers, such as ibuprofen, are often effective in managing this cramping.

3. **Nausea and Vomiting**: Some women may experience nausea or vomiting after taking mifepristone. These symptoms are more commonly associated with pregnancy and the body's hormonal changes rather than the drug itself. Nausea is generally mild and temporary, but in some cases, anti-nausea medication may be prescribed to alleviate the discomfort.

4. **Diarrhea**: Diarrhea is a less common but possible side effect. It may occur due to the body's response to mifepristone or misoprostol, particularly when the latter is taken orally. This side effect is usually mild and resolves on its own without the need for medical intervention.

5. **Fatigue**: Some women report feeling tired or fatigued after taking mifepristone. This fatigue may be related to the body's response to the drug or to the overall stress of undergoing a medical abortion. Rest and adequate hydration can help manage this side effect.

6. **Headache and Dizziness**: Headache and dizziness are also reported as common side effects. These symptoms are generally mild and can be managed with rest and over-the-counter pain relief if necessary.

While these side effects are common, they are typically short-lived and resolve as the body completes the abortion process. Most women can manage these symptoms at home with the support of a healthcare provider, and they do not usually require medical intervention.

4.2 Rare but Serious Side Effects

Although mifepristone is generally safe, there are rare but serious side effects that can occur. These side effects require immediate medical attention, as they can be life-threatening if left untreated. Some of the rare but serious side effects include:

1. **Severe Bleeding**: While bleeding is a normal part of the abortion process, in rare cases, it can become excessive. This condition, known as hemorrhage, may require medical intervention, such as a blood transfusion or surgical procedure, to stop the bleeding.

Women who experience soaking through two or more pads per hour for two consecutive hours, or who pass large clots, should seek medical attention immediately.

2. **Infection**: Although rare, an infection can occur if the uterus does not completely expel the pregnancy tissue, or if bacteria enter the uterus during the abortion process. Symptoms of infection may include fever, chills, severe abdominal pain, foul-smelling vaginal discharge, and prolonged heavy bleeding. Infections require prompt treatment with antibiotics and, in some cases, surgical intervention to remove any remaining tissue.

3. **Incomplete Abortion**: In some cases, the abortion may be incomplete, meaning that some pregnancy tissue remains in the uterus after taking mifepristone and misoprostol. This can lead to prolonged bleeding, infection, and continued symptoms of pregnancy. A follow-up appointment with a healthcare provider is essential to confirm that the abortion is complete. If the abortion is incomplete, additional doses of misoprostol or a surgical procedure may be necessary.

4. **Allergic Reactions**: Although extremely rare, some individuals may have an allergic reaction to mifepristone or misoprostol. Symptoms of an allergic

reaction may include rash, itching, swelling (especially of the face, tongue, or throat), severe dizziness, and difficulty breathing. An allergic reaction requires immediate medical attention, and the patient should be treated with appropriate antihistamines or other emergency interventions.

4.3 Contraindications

Mifepristone is not suitable for everyone, and there are certain contraindications that must be considered before its use. Contraindications refer to specific conditions or factors that make the use of mifepristone unsafe or inappropriate. Key contraindications include:

1. **Ectopic Pregnancy**: Mifepristone is contraindicated in women with an ectopic pregnancy, where the embryo implants outside the uterus, usually in a fallopian tube. Since mifepristone is ineffective in treating ectopic pregnancies, these must be addressed surgically or with other medical interventions to prevent life-threatening complications.

2. **Chronic Adrenal Failure**: Mifepristone is contraindicated in individuals with chronic adrenal

failure (Addison's disease), as the drug can block cortisol receptors, exacerbating the condition and leading to adrenal insufficiency, which is a medical emergency.

3. **Long-Term Corticosteroid Therapy**: Patients on long-term corticosteroid therapy, such as for autoimmune diseases or asthma, should not take mifepristone due to its potential to interfere with the effectiveness of corticosteroids, possibly leading to adrenal insufficiency.

4. **Coagulopathy or Anticoagulant Use**: Women with bleeding disorders, such as coagulopathy, or those taking anticoagulant medications (blood thinners) are at an increased risk of severe bleeding during a medical abortion and should not use mifepristone.

5. **IUD in Place**: Mifepristone should not be used by women who have an intrauterine device (IUD) in place, as the presence of the IUD can increase the risk of infection and other complications. The IUD should be removed before the administration of mifepristone.

6. **Allergy to Mifepristone or Misoprostol**: Patients with known hypersensitivity to mifepristone, misoprostol, or any component of these medications should avoid their use to prevent allergic reactions.

4.4 Interactions with Other Medications

Mifepristone can interact with other medications, which may alter its effectiveness or increase the risk of adverse effects. It is important for patients to inform their healthcare provider of all medications they are taking, including prescription drugs, over-the-counter medications, and dietary supplements. Some key drug interactions include:

1. **Corticosteroids**: As mentioned earlier, mifepristone can block the effects of corticosteroids, which are commonly used to treat inflammation and autoimmune conditions. Patients on long-term corticosteroid therapy should avoid mifepristone or be closely monitored by their healthcare provider.

2. **Anticoagulants**: Mifepristone can increase the risk of bleeding, particularly when taken with anticoagulants such as warfarin, heparin, or aspirin. Patients taking these medications should discuss alternative options with their healthcare provider.

3. **Cytochrome P450 Enzyme Inhibitors/Inducers**: Mifepristone is metabolized by the liver's cytochrome P450 enzyme system. Drugs that inhibit or induce these

enzymes, such as ketoconazole (an antifungal) or rifampin (an antibiotic), can affect the levels of mifepristone in the blood, potentially altering its effectiveness or increasing side effects.

4. **Nonsteroidal Anti-Inflammatory Drugs (NSAIDs)**: While NSAIDs like ibuprofen are often recommended to manage pain during a medical abortion, they should be used cautiously and under the guidance of a healthcare provider, as they may increase the risk of gastrointestinal bleeding.

5. **Herbal Supplements**: Some herbal supplements, particularly those that affect hormone levels or liver enzymes (e.g., St. John's Wort), can interact with mifepristone and should be discussed with a healthcare provider before use.

4.5 Safety Considerations

The safety of mifepristone, particularly in the context of medical abortion, is well-established when used according to approved guidelines. However, several safety considerations are important to ensure the best possible outcomes:

1. **Medical Supervision**: While mifepristone can be taken at home, it should be done under the supervision of a qualified healthcare provider. This ensures that the patient is a suitable candidate for medical abortion, that they understand the procedure, and that they have access to medical care if complications arise.

2. **Follow-Up Care**: A follow-up appointment is crucial to confirm that the abortion is complete and that there are no complications, such as an incomplete abortion or infection. This typically involves a physical examination or ultrasound 7 to 14 days after taking the medication.

3. **Emergency Plan**: Patients should be aware of the signs of serious complications, such as heavy bleeding, severe pain, or signs of infection, and have a plan in place for accessing emergency care if needed. Healthcare providers should provide clear instructions on when and how to seek help.

4. **Informed Consent**: Before taking mifepristone, patients should receive comprehensive counseling about the procedure, potential risks, side effects, and alternatives. Informed consent is essential to ensure that the patient fully understands the process and is making an informed decision.

5. **Emotional Support**: Undergoing a medical abortion can be an emotionally challenging experience for some women. Access to emotional support, whether through counseling services, support groups, or a trusted healthcare provider, can help women cope with the emotional aspects of the procedure.

CHAPTER 5

FREQUENTLY ASKED QUESTIONS

5.1 What Happens If You Take Mifepristone Outside of the Recommended Time Frame?

Mifepristone is most effective when taken within the first 10 weeks of pregnancy, which is calculated as 70 days from the first day of your last menstrual period. This is the time frame during which the drug has been extensively studied and shown to have the highest efficacy for pregnancy termination. Taking mifepristone outside of this recommended time frame can lead to several potential issues.

1. **Decreased Effectiveness**: The effectiveness of mifepristone decreases as pregnancy progresses beyond 10 weeks. After this period, the success rate of a medical abortion with mifepristone and misoprostol drops, increasing the likelihood of an incomplete abortion. An incomplete abortion means that not all of the pregnancy tissue is expelled, which can lead to complications such as heavy bleeding, infection, and

the need for surgical intervention to complete the process.

2. **Increased Risk of Complications**: As the pregnancy progresses, the size of the embryo or fetus increases, and the attachment to the uterine wall becomes more established. This can make the abortion process more difficult and increase the risk of complications such as severe bleeding and infection. Medical abortions performed after the 10-week mark should be done with caution and under close medical supervision.

3. **Need for Alternative Methods**: If you are beyond the 10-week mark, your healthcare provider may recommend alternative methods for pregnancy termination. These could include a higher dose or additional doses of misoprostol, or more commonly, a surgical abortion procedure such as vacuum aspiration or dilation and curettage (D&C), which are safe and effective options for later-term abortions.

4. **Legal and Regulatory Issues**: The use of mifepristone beyond 10 weeks may also be subject to legal and regulatory restrictions, depending on where you live. It is important to consult with a healthcare provider to understand the legal framework surrounding abortion in

your area and to ensure that you are following the recommended guidelines.

5.2 Can Mifepristone Be Used for Other Medical Conditions?

Yes, mifepristone has been approved for use in medical conditions beyond pregnancy termination, and its potential applications are being explored in various fields of medicine.

1. **Cushing's Syndrome**: Mifepristone is approved for the treatment of endogenous Cushing's syndrome, a condition characterized by an overproduction of cortisol by the adrenal glands. In this context, mifepristone acts as a glucocorticoid receptor antagonist, blocking the effects of cortisol. This helps alleviate the symptoms associated with Cushing's syndrome, such as high blood pressure, high blood sugar, and abnormal fat distribution. The dosage for Cushing's syndrome differs from that used in pregnancy termination and is tailored to the patient's specific needs.

2. **Uterine Fibroids**: Mifepristone has been studied as a treatment for uterine fibroids, which are non-cancerous

growths in the uterus that can cause heavy menstrual bleeding, pelvic pain, and other symptoms. Research suggests that mifepristone can shrink fibroids and reduce symptoms, although it is not yet widely approved for this use. Further studies are ongoing to determine its long-term efficacy and safety in treating fibroids.

3. **Endometriosis**: There is some evidence that mifepristone may be beneficial in treating endometriosis, a condition in which tissue similar to the lining of the uterus grows outside the uterus, causing pain and infertility. Mifepristone's ability to block progesterone may help reduce the growth of endometrial tissue and alleviate symptoms, but more research is needed to confirm its effectiveness and establish guidelines for its use in this condition.

4. **Breast Cancer**: Mifepristone has shown promise in preclinical studies as a potential treatment for certain types of breast cancer, particularly those that are hormone receptor-positive. By blocking the effects of progesterone, mifepristone may inhibit the growth of hormone-dependent tumors. However, this application is still experimental, and more research is required

before mifepristone can be recommended as a standard treatment for breast cancer.

5.3 What Should You Expect After Taking Mifepristone?

After taking mifepristone, especially as part of a medical abortion regimen, there are several things you can expect to happen as the drug takes effect.

1. **Initial Effects**: In the first 24 to 48 hours after taking mifepristone, you may not notice any significant changes. The drug works by blocking the hormone progesterone, which is necessary to maintain pregnancy. Without progesterone, the lining of the uterus begins to break down, and the pregnancy stops developing.

2. **Bleeding and Cramping**: The most noticeable effects usually begin after taking the second medication, misoprostol, which is typically taken 24 to 48 hours after mifepristone. Misoprostol causes the uterus to contract, leading to cramping and bleeding as the pregnancy tissue is expelled. The bleeding can range from light spotting to heavy, period-like bleeding with

clots. This is a normal part of the abortion process and usually lasts for several hours.

3. **Duration of Symptoms**: Cramping and bleeding can continue for several days to weeks, with the heaviest bleeding occurring within the first few hours after taking misoprostol. Some women may experience light bleeding or spotting for up to four weeks after the procedure. Other side effects, such as nausea, vomiting, diarrhea, and fatigue, may also occur but are generally mild and temporary.

4. **Emotional Response**: The emotional response to a medical abortion can vary widely. Some women may feel relief, while others may experience a range of emotions, including sadness, guilt, or anxiety. It is important to seek emotional support if needed and to talk to a healthcare provider or counselor if you are struggling with your feelings after the procedure.

5. **Follow-Up**: A follow-up visit with your healthcare provider is typically scheduled 7 to 14 days after taking mifepristone and misoprostol. This visit is important to confirm that the abortion is complete and that there are no complications. Your provider may perform an ultrasound or a physical examination to ensure that all

pregnancy tissue has been expelled and that your uterus is returning to its normal state.

5.4 Are There Alternatives to Mifepristone for Early Pregnancy Termination?

Yes, there are several alternatives to mifepristone for early pregnancy termination. The choice of method depends on factors such as the stage of pregnancy, personal preference, medical history, and access to care.

1. **Misoprostol Alone**: In some cases, misoprostol can be used alone to induce abortion, especially in settings where mifepristone is not available. Misoprostol is less effective when used on its own compared to when it is used in combination with mifepristone, but it can still be a viable option. The success rate for a misoprostol-only abortion is slightly lower, and it may require multiple doses or a longer time frame to complete the process.

2. **Surgical Abortion**: Surgical abortion is another option for early pregnancy termination. The most common methods are vacuum aspiration and dilation and curettage (D&C). These procedures are performed by a

healthcare provider in a clinical setting and involve the physical removal of pregnancy tissue from the uterus. Surgical abortion is highly effective and is typically completed in one visit, with immediate confirmation that the pregnancy has been terminated.

3. **Expectant Management**: In some cases, expectant management, or waiting for a miscarriage to occur naturally, may be an option for early pregnancy termination, particularly in cases of early fetal demise or non-viable pregnancy. This approach involves monitoring the pregnancy and allowing the body to expel the pregnancy tissue on its own without medical intervention. However, this option may not be suitable for everyone, and the decision should be made in consultation with a healthcare provider.

4. **Methotrexate and Misoprostol**: Another alternative, though less commonly used, is the combination of methotrexate and misoprostol. Methotrexate is a drug that stops the growth of rapidly dividing cells, including those of the pregnancy. It is used in combination with misoprostol to induce abortion. This method is less commonly used due to the availability of more effective options, but it may be considered in certain circumstances, such as in early ectopic pregnancies.

5.5 How to Access Mifepristone

Access to mifepristone varies depending on where you live, as it is subject to different legal and regulatory restrictions around the world. Here are some general guidelines on how to access mifepristone:

1. **Consult a Healthcare Provider**: The first step to accessing mifepristone is to consult with a healthcare provider who is qualified to prescribe the medication. This could be a doctor, nurse practitioner, or another licensed medical professional. They will assess your eligibility for a medical abortion, provide counseling on the procedure, and prescribe the medication if appropriate.
2. **Telemedicine Services**: In some regions, mifepristone can be prescribed and accessed through telemedicine services. This allows you to consult with a healthcare provider remotely, receive a prescription, and have the medication delivered to your home. Telemedicine is becoming increasingly common, especially in areas where access to abortion services is limited. It is important to ensure that the service you use is

legitimate and operates within the legal framework of your country or state.

3. **Pharmacies**: Once prescribed, mifepristone can be obtained from certain pharmacies. In some countries, the drug is only available through specialized clinics or healthcare providers, while in others, it may be available at retail pharmacies. Your healthcare provider will guide you on where to fill your prescription.

4. **Planned Parenthood and Abortion Clinics**: In the United States and some other countries, organizations like Planned Parenthood and other abortion clinics offer mifepristone as part of their services. These clinics provide comprehensive care, including counseling, the administration of the medication, and follow-up care. They can also offer support and resources if you encounter any issues during the process.

5. **Legal Considerations**: It is crucial to be aware of the legal status of mifepristone in your region. In some countries and states, access to abortion, including medical abortion with mifepristone, may be restricted by law. In such cases, seeking care from a licensed provider who operates within the legal framework is essential to avoid legal consequences.

6. **Financial Assistance**: If cost is a concern, there may be financial assistance programs available to help cover the cost of mifepristone and related services. Organizations that support reproductive health and rights often provide resources or referrals to programs that can help reduce the financial burden.

Accessing mifepristone safely and legally is essential to ensure that you receive the care and support you need during a medical abortion. By consulting with a qualified healthcare provider and following the appropriate guidelines, you can make informed decisions about your reproductive health.

CHAPTER 6

CONCLUSION

6.1 Summary of Key Points

Mifepristone, also known as RU-486, is a medication that plays a crucial role in the medical management of early pregnancy termination. It is widely recognized for its effectiveness in inducing abortion within the first 10 weeks of pregnancy. The use of mifepristone, often in combination with misoprostol, provides a non-invasive alternative to surgical abortion, offering women more autonomy and privacy in managing their reproductive health.

In **Chapter 1**, we discussed the **Overview of Early Pregnancy Termination** and introduced mifepristone, covering its history, development, and relevance. Mifepristone, by inhibiting the hormone progesterone, effectively halts the progression of pregnancy, allowing for a controlled and predictable process of termination. Its development has been pivotal in expanding the options available for women seeking to terminate a pregnancy, particularly in the early stages.

Chapter 2 focused on how mifepristone works, including its **Mechanism of Action, Effectiveness, and Time Frame for Usage**. The drug's ability to block progesterone is central to its function, leading to the detachment of the gestational sac from the uterine lining, followed by the administration of misoprostol to induce uterine contractions and expel the pregnancy tissue. Mifepristone's effectiveness, especially when used within the recommended time frame, is well-documented, with success rates exceeding 95% in early pregnancy termination.

In **Chapter 3**, we explored the **Usage Guidelines** for mifepristone, including indications for use, dosage instructions, and what to do if a dose is missed. These guidelines are essential for ensuring the safe and effective use of the drug, particularly given its powerful effects on the body. Following the prescribed protocol and adhering to medical supervision are critical components of a successful medical abortion.

Chapter 4 covered the **Side Effects and Safety** of mifepristone, detailing common side effects such as bleeding, cramping, nausea, and rare but serious risks like severe bleeding and infection. We also discussed contraindications, drug interactions, and safety considerations, emphasizing the importance of medical supervision and follow-up care to minimize risks and ensure the procedure's success.

In **Chapter 5**, we addressed **Frequently Asked Questions**, including what happens if mifepristone is taken outside the recommended time frame, its potential uses for other medical conditions, and alternatives for early pregnancy termination. We also provided guidance on how to access mifepristone, which varies depending on regional legal frameworks and healthcare systems.

6.2 Final Recommendations

Based on the comprehensive exploration of mifepristone's role in early pregnancy termination and its broader medical applications, several key recommendations emerge for those considering its use or involved in its administration.

1. **Adhere to the Recommended Time Frame**: Mifepristone is most effective when used within the first 10 weeks of pregnancy. Patients should be aware of this critical window and seek medical consultation as early as possible if considering a medical abortion. Taking the medication outside of this period may reduce its effectiveness and increase the risk of complications, making it essential to follow medical guidance closely.

2. **Ensure Medical Supervision**: While mifepristone offers the convenience of a medical abortion that can be initiated at home, it is imperative that this process is conducted under the supervision of a qualified

healthcare provider. Medical supervision ensures that the patient is a suitable candidate for mifepristone, that the medication is used correctly, and that any potential complications are promptly addressed.

3. **Understand the Side Effects and Risks**: Patients should be fully informed about the possible side effects and risks associated with mifepristone. This includes common symptoms like bleeding and cramping, as well as rarer but more serious risks such as infection or incomplete abortion. Knowing what to expect and when to seek medical attention is crucial for a safe and successful outcome.

4. **Follow-Up Care is Essential**: A follow-up visit is a critical component of the medical abortion process. This visit ensures that the abortion is complete and that there are no lingering complications. It also provides an opportunity for patients to discuss any concerns or emotional responses they may have experienced. Skipping this step can lead to undetected complications and potential long-term health issues.

5. **Consider Alternatives If Necessary**: For those who are not suitable candidates for mifepristone or who are beyond the recommended time frame, alternative methods of pregnancy termination should be discussed

with a healthcare provider. Surgical abortion procedures like vacuum aspiration or dilation and curettage (D&C) are safe and effective alternatives that may be more appropriate in certain cases.

6. **Access Mifepristone Safely and Legally**: Access to mifepristone is regulated in many regions, and it is important to obtain the medication through legal and safe channels. This may involve consulting a licensed healthcare provider, utilizing telemedicine services where available, or visiting a reputable clinic such as those operated by organizations like Planned Parenthood. Patients should be wary of unregulated sources or illegal channels, as these can pose significant health risks.

7. **Seek Emotional and Psychological Support**: Undergoing a medical abortion can be an emotionally complex experience. Patients should be encouraged to seek support from counselors, support groups, or trusted individuals in their lives. Emotional well-being is an important aspect of overall health, and addressing it can help in coping with the abortion process and its aftermath.

8. **Stay Informed About Legal and Regulatory Changes**: The legal landscape surrounding abortion is

subject to change, particularly in countries and states where access to reproductive healthcare is a contentious issue. Patients and healthcare providers should stay informed about any changes in laws and regulations that might affect access to mifepristone and other abortion services. Advocacy for reproductive rights and access to safe abortion care remains crucial in many parts of the world.

9. **Education and Advocacy**: Healthcare providers should engage in ongoing education about the latest developments in medical abortion and the use of mifepristone. Additionally, advocacy for improved access to safe abortion services, including the availability of mifepristone, is essential for ensuring that all individuals have the ability to make informed choices about their reproductive health.

FINALLY, mifepristone has revolutionized the options available for early pregnancy termination, offering a safe, effective, and non-invasive alternative to surgical abortion. Its benefits extend beyond pregnancy termination, with potential applications in treating conditions like Cushing's syndrome, uterine fibroids, and possibly hormone-sensitive cancers. However, its use requires careful adherence to medical guidelines, an understanding of the associated risks, and access to appropriate follow-up care. By following these recommendations, patients and healthcare providers can ensure that mifepristone is used safely and effectively, empowering women to make informed decisions about their reproductive health.